1

purchase your own copy. Thank you for

valuing the author's work.

Please leave feedback on the website from which you purchased this book. We authors truly do appreciate our readers and love to connect with you.

Chapter 1 – Introduction

This book is a no nonsense guide to getting into physician assistant school. It was written under the assumption that you, the reader, have already decided to become a physician assistant, have already researched the profession and the schools you'd like to attend, and now just need the exact information to guide you to getting into the school. This book is short, concise, and packed full of useful information. If you are looking for a book full of hundreds of pages of fluff, please choose a different book. And without further ado, please enjoy reading "BE A PA, How to get into physician assistant school without a flawless application".

Becoming a PA is no small task. The best time to decide to become a PA is early in your educational career. It is better to decide to become a PA before you start your undergrad associate's degree. This is because the entry requirements for physician assistant school are different than that of other medical professions.

Therefore, the earlier that you decide to become a PA the better. If you want to get a head start, decide to become a PA in high school. But even if you decide to become a PA later in life, it is a very doable task. I know many PAs that decided to become a physician assistant after they had already had careers of their own.

In fact, the physician assistant that I shadowed the most was first an electrician before he became a PA. But then he hurt his back and could no longer work as an electrician. So he decided go back to school and become a physician assistant. And although the physician assistant career causes him to either be on his feet for long periods of time or sitting in a chair for long periods of time and can be harmful on his back, it is still much easier on his back than manual labor.

In this book I have outlined the many steps that I took to get into PA school even though I have a less than a flawless application. It took very hard work and a lot of dedication, but eventually I got my goal. In fact, I got into the exact school that I wanted to.

So in this book I will detail the steps that I took to get into assistant school.

It all started the day that I was outside playing football. Unfortunately, I made a very stupid mistake. But that's what life is about isn't it? Life's full of mistakes that we learn from, correct, and then turn the lessons into success. This mistake, however, gave me a scar for life... Literally!

On this day, even though the sun was not shining because it was completely cloud covered, I decided to wear sunglasses. Of course we were playing flag football and not tackle, but that did not save me. We were playing five on five organized flag football. My buddy, the quarterback, took the snap and I ran a quick out route to his left. He threw the ball to me low and behind me. As I reached back to catch the football, I lost my footing and fell to the ground. As I was getting back up, a defender, who was running up to pull my flag, accidentally kneed me in the forehead.

His knee hit the sunglasses so hard that it split my forehead open. That is the day that I will never forget. It did not hurt as much as it bled. Another friend of mine's wife, handed me a shirt to stop the bleeding and drove me to the hospital.

When I got there, there was not much of a wait. About 15 minutes after I was triaged, I was lying on the bed and a physician assistant was suturing my wound. It took a total of 36 stitches to completely seal the wound, twelve inside stitches and twenty-four outside stitches. The PA who stitched me up kept asking me if I needed more lidocaine. I told him that I was more concerned with scar than the pain since the wound was right on my forehead. He laughed and said that he would try his best to minimize the scar.

I must say that the physician assistant who sutured my wound did a wonderful job. Most people, even if they notice the scar, do not say anything about it. Unless of course, I bring it up first. It is noticeable but not upon first glance. That is what I wanted.

That experience is a major reason why I wanted to become a physician assistant. But, I wish it would have happened earlier in my life. But I have no regrets.

The following book is going to outline the limbs of the tree that sprung from this little seed of experience that propelled me into physician assistant school.

Soon after this experience, I looked up physician assistant schools on Google. I printed out the prerequisites for three schools in my state. Although I researched three schools in my state, I chose one to actually attend. But I would have been happy to be accepted into any of them.

The following seven chapters are going to describe the seven steps that I took to get into physician assistant school. Mind you, I already did not have a quality application. I had a lot of work to do. The seven steps are as follows: focus on your undergraduate study and make sure you have a high grade point average (GPA), make sure that you make great connections so that you can have plenty of shadowing hours and awesome references, study your butt off for the GRE exam, make sure that you have the CASPA filled out correctly and write an astonishing essay (which I will tell you how to do), research fully the interview process and make sure you are completely prepared for it, and finally, what you need to do after the interview to ensure that a spot in a physician assistant school is reserved for you.

And make sure that you read to the very end and do not skip any section because at the end, I've included an amazing bonus.

Chapter 2 – Undergraduate

The reason why I said in the introduction that it is better to decide to be a physician assistant early in your educational career is so that you can wipe out all of the prerequisites early in your undergraduate education.

Unfortunately for me, I did not decide to become a physician assistant until after I had already received an Associate's degree. Even though this Associates degree was in medicine so to speak, or at least science-based, it still did not prepare me as far as undergraduate education is concerned for entry into the physician field. Therefore, when I went to get my Bachelor's degree and told my counselor that I wanted to become a physician assistant, she looked blankly at me, and gave me a condescending stare, and told me that I had a lot of work to do. I left her office filling less than encourage.

I had a GPA of roughly 3.12 and actually failed one class. I will speak more about the class that I failed during chapter 6 on the interview. But for now, I had a less than stellar GPA, two year's worth of classes that I still needed to take, and the class, microbiology, that I had to retake because the one that I took for undergrad was only a 2000 level class and they required a 3000 level class.

But I did not give up. I immediately enrolled for my Bachelor's degree and began taking classes. Unfortunately, I made another mistake. I took a class that I thought satisfied a certain criteria. But after I took the class, that criteria was not satisfied. This mistake alone cost me an entire semester.

And let's not forget the semesters I wasted during my Associates degree training while I was out partying and chasing girls rather than focusing on my studies. I worked full time all through my undergrad including all through my Bachelor's program. But I still could have taken more classes each semester. But instead I decided to go out with my friends and party. This was a big mistake. And my caution to you is to focus on your education early and worry about partying once you're in your career.

So my education was already pushed back roughly 4 years due in part because of my immature nature and in part because of my one mistake choosing a class. But these were not my biggest mistake. My biggest mistake is continuing to party while I was trying to attain my Bachelor's degree. I was still an immature kid.

This partying lead me to having silver bracelets on my wrists and a public record. No I did not get into a fight and no I did not get a felony. What I got was a misdemeanor known as driving while under the influence (DUI) of alcohol. Yes that was my mistake.

And yes, this mistake cured my party disease. It cost me roughly $10,000 because I hired an attorney to fight my case. First, all I wanted was a consult but she convinced me that my case was strong and that the officers were not in any right to hold me. I literally had to sit on the side of the road after the officer asked me to move my car and wait for the arresting officer to show up and perform the sobriety test.

I obviously failed this test and he immediately slapped handcuffs on me, threw me in the back of his cop car, and took me straight to jail. I was fingerprinted, mug "shotted", and placed into a holding cell for eight hours, which is the standard time to allow your body to process the alcohol in your system.

Luckily for me, one of the officers sitting at the desk called my parents to bail me out. I got out that afternoon and was fully ashamed of myself. I thanked my parents for bailing me out but I'm sure I did not speak with conviction. The embarrassment was just too great.

I was also lucky in the fact that a DUI is a misdemeanor and not a felony. But this misdemeanor not only set me back $10,000 but also another semester in school. My attorney took many months of fighting my case before she got my conviction reduced to reckless driving. But I still had to go through all the reprimanding that is required for those convicted of DUI as ordered by the judge in accordance with my plea deal.

The punishment included $500 to bail me out, 50 hours of community service, attending a two day DUI class, 12 sessions of psychological addiction counseling (kind of like AA), my license suspended for a month before I got my work permit and then another month before I got my actual license back, and a session where we had to sit and watch videos of people speaking about their loved ones who were killed by a drunk driver.

At the time, I thought the punishment was excessive. But in retrospect, I thought it was fair. I will never make that mistake again.

I digress, but I had to tell you about my story and why I am so pushy about focusing on your education when you are in your undergrad. I could have been completely derailed from my plans. But again, I knew what I wanted and I did not quit.

So with that said, don't mess around during your undergrad. Make sure you keep your GPA high because competition is great and is becoming greater over time. The faculty at physician assistant schools have hundreds of applications they must read and they only pick the best ones to interview. So you must set yourself apart from the others.

Of course one thing about having a less than flawless application that can help you stand out is your ability to bounce back from adversity. Make sure you feature this during your application process because when you are in physician assistant school, there will be many challenges and you will have to face a lot of adversity.

It is recommended to have a GPA of 3.5 or greater to be considered competitive. After I got my Bachelor's degree, I brought my GPA up from 3.12 to 3.39. This does not seem astonishing, but due to the number of credit hours I had already accumulated, this feat still amazes me today. Again, as you can see, my GPA was less than outstanding.

If you do have a GPA of 3.5 or higher, you will have less to overcome. But having a GPA of less than 3.5 is not a warrant for failure. Getting into physician assistant school is still a very feasible option. So do not be discouraged.

By not delaying your undergraduate education and by taking a full slate of classes and keeping your GPA high, you set yourself up to be in the best possible position to be admitted to a physician assistant school. Naturally, this is not earth shattering knowledge. But I still feel the need to reiterate that your undergraduate education is very important once you decide on your career path.

Another tip for your undergrad education is to not take the easy route. Physician assistant school will not do you any favors. The classes are hard, the hours are long, and the pace is ridiculously fast. So do yourself a favor and challenge yourself during your undergrad by taking as many classes as you feel like you can handle, and as many hard classes as you can handle. When you have a choice to take an easy class or a hard class, always choose the hard class. This will make sure that you are prepared for and can handle physician assistant school.

Organic chemistry is the class that weeds out those students who are either not ready for graduate school, or who are not really made for the medical field. And organic chemistry is a joke compared to what you will face while you are in physician assistant school. It's not necessarily that the material is hard, but more so the pace of the education and the way the professors expect you to interpret and apply the information.

The harder you push yourself in undergrad, the more you will be prepared for your physician assistant graduate studies. So go for the biomedical degree rather than the health science degree. And do not fret for your hard work will pay off.

Next we will discuss making connections with physician assistants and accumulating shadowing hours and letters of references.

Chapter 3 - Connections

Now that you have your undergraduate
degree, both Associates and Bachelors, it is
time to start making strong connections with
physician assistants. In fact, I would
recommend making these connections along
the way as you are getting your undergraduate
degrees. If you can get shadowing hours
during your undergrad, this will not only
prepare you for what you are going to face
during your career, but it will also save you a
lot of time once you graduate since you will
already have tons of shadowing hours and
letters of recommendation as you prepare to
take your GRE exam.

So, how do you go about attaining shadowing
hours?

The answer to this question is actually quite
simple. Just call up any of your local
emergency rooms and ask to speak to a PA.
Once a PA comes onto the phone, simply
and respectfully tell them that you are an
aspiring physician assistant and ask them if it

is okay with them if you do a few shadowing hours with them.

> **Example:** "Hi, my name is Nathaniel, and I am an aspiring physician assistant. I am currently taking my undergraduate studies but would love to attain some shadowing hours because I know that they are very important. I'm calling around to see if I can find a physician assistant to shadow. Is it okay if I come down during your next shift so that we can meet and maybe work something out?"

Or, if you know somebody who works in a hospital, regardless of their position, ask them to go down to the emergency room and ask a physician assistant if a friend of theirs can shadow them. This way you have the benefit of an insider. This works out better just like getting a date with someone works out better if you know someone who knows the other person rather than approaching them cold. Having someone approach a physician assistant for you is called a warm approach rather than a cold approach or a cold call, which is much more effective.

I was lucky here to. I actually worked at a hospital in the medical records department. In this way, when I went down to the emergency department in my hospital, since I worked there, the physician assistants were less on the defensive. And I must point out also that shadowing a physician assistant is a must. I first shadowed a physician and during my interview, the interviewers frowned upon the fact that I had not shadowed a physician assistant. It is okay to shadow a nurse practitioner, a physician, a radiologist, etc... But make sure that the majority of your shadowing is done with a physician assistant. Shadowing those aforementioned medical professionals will allow you an amazing benefit during the interview process. This benefit will be divulged more deeply in chapter 6.

Regardless of your method, you need to shadow and make connections with a physician assistant. While you shadow the physician assistant, bring a pad and a pencil or pen so you can write down ideas. It is okay and preferred that you ask questions while you are shadowing and write down the answers. This shows that you have interest in the career and helps you build rapport with the physician assistant whom you are shadowing. The more you are liked by the physician assistant you are shadowing, the more they will be willing to write you a letter of recommendation.

Furthermore, it is also recommended that you shadow physician assistants at multiple locations and multiple departments. For example, you would like to get shadowing experience in the emergency room, and an orthopedic office, and obstetrics, and in a mother baby unit. The benefit of shadowing in a hospital is you have access to every one of these units and more. I'm not saying that the previously mentioned specialties are preferred, I just use them as an example to emphasize that it is best to be diversified with your shadowing hours.

CASPA requires three letters of recommendation and one of them has to be a physician assistant. So again, it is okay if you shadow and get letters of recommendation from other professions than the physician assistant as long as at least one letter of recommendation is from a physician assistant. But it is preferred that at least two are from physician assistants.

Now, once you have a physician assistant shadowing opportunity set up for you, make sure that you call them ahead of time and ask them for the correct dress code. Some places may just require you to wear scrubs, some may require suits, and some may require some kind of lab coat. But make sure you get this settled before your first day so you do not look silly when you show up. And make sure that you have comfortable shoes because you may be on your feet quite a bit.

It is also recommended that you bring with you a stethoscope so that if the opportunity presents itself, you can listen to heartbeats, lung sounds, and belly sounds while you shadow. There are a few things that you are allowed to do but your experience will be limited.

I, for example, was allowed to assist splinting a patient's arm, listened to a child's breath sounds, and listen to numerous heart beats. I was also allowed to speak with the patients, asked them questions, and consulted with a physician assistant to practice my diagnosing skills. You will see as you shadow that often cases repeat themselves. And if you pay attention, you will get good at diagnosing the patients.

> **Tip:** While you are in physician assistant school, make sure that you do not refer to the patient as "my patient". PAs frown upon that saying because the patient is the physician's patient not the physician assistant's.

Another perk of having great rapport with a physician assistant whom you're shadowing is that you will be able to call them once you are in physician assistant school and ask him or her questions and gain guidance. And trust me when I say you will need it. PA school is tough.

Let me take this time now to reassure you that although PA school is tough, it is very passable. I just don't want you to walk into PA school thinking that you have it handled because you will struggle and they know you struggle. But if you put your mind to it, you can do it. And you would not be reading this book if you have not already decided that this is what you want to do.

In closing this chapter, I will say that shadowing physician assistants is more important than working around them. You do not have to be a scribe, nurse, or emergency technician to become a physician assistant. Although these jobs do help.

Now that we have received our undergraduate degree with a 3.5 or greater GPA, attained shadowing hours and letters of recommendation, we now must face the daunting task of passing the GRE exam.

Chapter 4 - GRE

This exam, unfortunately, is not applicable to the physician assistant degree. I, for one, do not understand why we had to take this exam. This exam is composed of five or six sections. These sections include: two math sections, two verbal sections, and one or two writing sections. One of the sections, which could be verbal, math, and or writing sections, does not count. This experimental section is used for editing future exams.

The GRE is designed to trick you and not to test your knowledge. This is the fact no matter what anyone tells you. The only reason why they would design the test the way they do is to try to deceive you.

The math section is not exactly hard. But the way the formulas are written can make the math hard. Instead of a straight up question such as X squared equals nine, they give you something that looks like this:

Example: A   B

x^2 | $x - 4$

Which is bigger?

The above equation comparison is a prime example of how the GRE is formatted. This is a very easy example. The examples on exam will be much harder. The key here is to plug in numbers. The numbers to plug-in are as follows: -2, -1, 0, 1, 2, and a +/- fraction such as -1/2 and +1/2. The reason why you use two digits negative and two digits positive is because the number 1 can be deceiving just as 0 can be deceiving.

For example, one squared equals itself, but two squared equals four, and zero squared also equals itself. Remember to plug-in these numbers as you solve equations. In the above equation, the first answer choice (A) would be correct because no matter what number you plug-in for the X in the equation on the right, it will be smaller than the answer to the equation on the left. And the answer on the left can never be negative.

However, often the answer will be cannot be determined.

Example: A   B

$$x^2 \quad | \quad x^3$$

Which is bigger?

The answer to above question is cannot be determined because, as you can see if you plug-in the above recommended numbers, sometimes A will be bigger and sometimes B will be bigger.

I would be remiss if I did not mention that the GRE **will** have many tricky sentences and words. Watch for phrases like X is a non-negative integer, which is bigger, which is smaller, and they are equal. These may not seem tricky but make sure that you read the question fully before starting to determine the answer. And make sure that you read the answer choices correctly and read all of them before marking your final answer.

You will also encounter equations such as this:

Example: Which of the following is greater than X, where -1 < x < 1

1. x^2
2. 1-x

26

3. $\sqrt{x}$
4. $x^3 - x^2$
5. $x^4 - 4x$

Make sure you plug in your answer choices for each numbered answer choices (-½ , 0, ½). This will be a tedious project but must be done. However, for questions like this that take a long time, I'd recommend marking an answer (as a guess) and then marking the question for review and then going to the next question. Once you finish the math section, then go back and review all the marked answers. This way, you won't spend all of your time trying to answer a single question and end up having to Christmas tree the rest of the math section. And if you do not have time to go back and work out the problem, at least you have an answer marked. A blank answer is scored just like a wrong answer.

> **Tip:** When marking an answer, avoid using the scroll bar on the mouse to scroll down or you risk changing your answer. If you are addicted to using the scroll bar on the mouse to scroll down, practice clicking any blank spot

on the screen before scrolling down
until it becomes a habit. This will
prevent you from inadvertently
changing your answers.

For a more comprehensive review of the
math section of the GRE, pick yourself up a
comprehensive GRE guide. I prefer the
Princeton Review (no, I do not have an
endorsement deal with them). It is the book
that I used to study. And also use the Kaplan
online educational tool for more study
material and multiple practice exams.

During the exam, you will have at least one
pencil, at least one sheet of paper, a
calculator (probably an on-screen calculator
on the computer you are using to take the
exam), and headphones to block out noise.
Unfortunately for me, I was seated right by
the entry door and the noise blocking
headphones did not fit on my head. Every
few minutes someone would walk by the
door and it would disturb me. So if you get
seated by the door, make sure you at least
request to be moved to a different seat.

Now we will move to the verbal section. At the end of the GRE chapter, I will give you a comprehensive review of the GRE exam experience and what you need to do to prepare, including how to study and how much you need to study. But this is also going to be covered in your GRE review book.

The verbal section of the GRE is just as tricky, if not trickier, than the math section. Again, you will have two math sections and two verbal sections (or three of either verbal or math if you get these sections as your experimental section). The verbal section is tricky because there will be a lot of words that you do not know and sentences that are picked out of paragraphs for which there is no context. In these non-contextual sentences, you will need to plug-in words to complete the sentence or to make the sentences make sense. Often there will be one word that you can exclude right away. And then there will be two words that are so close and fit so perfectly that you will have to just flip a coin, figuratively speaking.

Studying for the GRE will cause you to learn words like cacophony, discordant, putrid, entelechy, and esoteric. If you do not know any of these words, go ahead right now and look them up and commit the definition to memory. I will give you one definition: Entelechy means to take potential and turn it into reality.

A tip with definitions: try to take the Webster's definition, or the definition you receive from your GRE comprehensive guide, and turn it into your own words. The GRE usually does not ask you many questions, or any questions at all, regarding the actual definition of the word. It tests you more on whether or not you actually know what the word is and how to use it. So by having your own definition, you can program your mind to actually know what the word is and how to use it.

The verbal section will have definitions, text completion, and reading comprehension questions. Yes, there will be definitions. But as I mentioned above, there will be less of these types of questions than the others.

Example: He did not understand John's _____ language and, therefore, did not know how to reply.

A. Discordant
B. Anomalous
C. Esoteric
D. Inchoate

That's how tricky some of the GRE questions can be. The good news is that not all of them are this hard. First you must know what each of the words means. If you do not know what a word means, but you know the other words do not fit, then pick the word you do not know. If there are two words you do not know, and the two that you do know do not fit, then pick the one you think is the best. But if you do not know a word and you know the words that you do know do not fit, do not sit there and dwell on the question for far too long. You have a limited number of minutes to complete each section, so use your time wisely.

Discordant means harsh or annoying in sound. Anomalous means different than the normal. Esoteric means understood by a select few or inside knowledge. And inchoate means incomplete or disorganized. From the outset, all of them except for the first choice seem like they fit. If his language is anomalous, esoteric, or inchoate, then his words could be misunderstood. So you are going to have to do a little reasoning. Since he did not know how to reply to John's language, then you can probably strike out inchoate because you can always ask the person to repeat what he says if it is not clear. So that leaves us with anomalous and esoteric. If something is anomalous that does not necessarily mean that it is hard to understand. It just means that someone uses language that is different than what someone else would normally use. So this could mean someone can use the word gigantic in a situation that you would normally use the word huge. But both of these words mean the same thing and are easily understood. Therefore esoteric, which actually means only understood by a few people, would be the most logical choice. And esoteric, C, is the correct choice.

Sentences will give you a little more information than this one did. But you will have a few questions like this on the GRE. Make sure that you reread the answer at least twice and reread the question at least twice so that you can pick out the keywords.

For a more comprehensive review of the verbal section of the GRE and for full list of words make sure you pick up a comprehensive GRE guide. If you need to, make flashcards of words and practice them daily. Remember, just because you know a word does not mean that you're going to remember it the next day. So as you move on to new words each day, make sure you review the words you remembered from the previous days.

When I took the GRE, there were also questions about the main idea and the theme of a paragraph. You will probably encounter a few questions like this as well. But there are not a ton. So as long as you practice what is written about in the comprehensive guide, you should be fine.

And the final section is the essay. Usually the essay is an opinionated question. But there are also some facts that must be included. So for example, the GRE will have a paragraph and you will be asked to reply to the paragraph either for it or against it.

The essay section is straightforward. As long as you know grammar and punctuation, this will be an easy task for you. So make sure you put some personality into your essay so that it will not be boring for those who read it. If you can affect someone's emotions, you will get a much better response. Even if your essay's quality is lacking, an emotional essay will more than make up for this limitation.

When I studied for the GRE, I studied for six weeks straight. I would get up early in the morning and go to the library before work. I did this for the first three weeks. For six days a week, I would study either math or verbal. I would switch the days so that I did not get burnt out. So on Monday, for example, I would study math. Then on Tuesday I would review what I studied on math and then study some verbal. And I would continue this rotation. After the first three weeks, I started studying more at home.

It is also good to take to exams each week to test your knowledge. But do not be discouraged if you are not getting the scores they want. It is good to retake exams each week as well. But make sure you leave at least two exams that have questions from each section that you absolutely do not take until two days before your exam. The reason why you take these exams two days before your real exam day and not the day before is because you need the day before to rest. You do not want to go into test day exhausted.

So make sure you study for the GRE, however you study, for at least six weeks before your exam. For the verbal section, if you need to, make flashcards. While you are studying the math section, make sure you use a simple calculator like the one you will have to use on the exam.

And when you study, make sure that you study when you're at your best. If you are a morning person, study in the morning. If you

are a night person, study at night. Review
your materials each day that you've studied
the day before so you do not forget it.
Remember, repetition is the mother of skill.

For the math, I just did the math sections in
the comprehensive GRE guide. For the
verbal, I memorize as many words as
possible in the amount of time that I was
given. Then I would take practice exams,
both on the computer (the CD that came
with the Princeton review and the Kaplan
website) and written by hand. I also set a
deadline and registered for the exam before I
started studying. By doing this, I put in
motion a study plan. If you do not register for
the exam, you risk wasting a lot of time and
not really studying because you'll feel like
you have plenty of time and you will not have
a sense of urgency. This is just my
recommendation: register for your test day
before you start studying.

So you've studied for six weeks, took
multiple practice exams, and now it is two
days before the exam. In the morning, take a
few hours and just review the material that
you've learned. Try not to learn new stuff at

this point. Then take a break and come back in the afternoon and take your two practice exams. Try to take the exams exactly how they are going to give them to you on the real test day. In fact, for the last two weeks of your study time try to take your practice exams exactly as they will give them to you on the real exam and at the exact time that you've registered for the real GRE exam. However, on this last day of practice exams, give yourself at least a half an hour between your two exams to allow your brain to rest.

By this time, you should be getting at least 80% or greater on your exams. The day before your exam, do not study during the day. Take the day off and relax. The evening before your exam, make sure you treat yourself to a good meal and have a little fun. You need to laugh the night before your exam and have a good time. But also make sure that you go to bed early so you get plenty of sleep. But before you go to bed, take a very quick review of your materials. You are not studying at this time. In fact, two days before your real GRE exam, you should go ahead and write up your review that you are going to review the next day. At this time it will be good to write down things that you probably do not know or think that you will easily forget. These are the things you should review the day before your exam.

If you are the type of person who has test anxiety, bring your study materials with you to the exam. You can study these materials in your car or outside of the test area before your scheduled time. But remember not to burn yourself out.

So now you are prepared. You took your two practice exams and got at least 80%. You want to bed and woke up the next day and had some fun. You reviewed the material that you wrote down so you won't forget. You reviewed them the night before the exam and had a good meal. You went to bed early and got plenty of sleep. And now you woke up otn his test day.

Have a healthy low carb high-protein breakfast. Make sure you wake up early enough to have plenty of time to eat, use the restroom, look up traffic and drive to the testing center, and review your study materials if you need to. Do not drink a lot fluids. You may get up to use the restroom during your exam but if you're still in a timed section and the time will continue to run.

> **Tip:** Set out your exam materials that you are going to bring with you on exam day the night before so they are already ready to go. And, on the morning of the exam, do not drink too much caffeine. It will make you jittery and will cause you to make little mistakes on the exam. Know your body!

When you arrive at the testing center, you will need your identification, proof of registration for the exam, and make sure that you are not wearing or bring in anything that will not fit in your locker that they give you. You cannot bring anything into the exam. They will make you pull out your pockets, scan you with a metal detector, make you take your belt and hat off, and please do not bring in your phone. Research the center where you will be taking the exam to get the full details of their rules and regulations.

So you turn in all your registration materials and fill out a short waiver and then they give you a key to a locker. This key is the only thing you are allowed to have in your pocket. Then they walk you into the little room right outside computer room where you will be taking your exam. They make sure that you do not have any material on you and a scan you down with a metal detector. They sign you in with the time and then walk you to a computer. This is where you can request a better computer if you do not like your location. They then sign you into the computer and tell you that you may be seated.

Then once you are seated, they give you verbal instructions or the instructions are written on the computer. You get a few minutes to get comfortable with the computer system. Then once you click start, the time starts. As mentioned before, they will give you a sheet of paper and a pencil or pen and the calculator will most likely be on the computer itself. You will also have a soundproof headphone set that you may put on your head if you'd like.

Every time you leave the test center, you must sign out with the time. And every time you re-enter the test center, you must sign in with the time. You may not take anything out of the test center except for the key to your locker.

When you are finally done with your exam, you get your scores right away, except for the written essay which is scored by a person. Your score is broken down into verbal and math sections. To be competitive for the PA programs, you must get a 300 or better. On my first and only try at the GRE, I received a 302; 151 verbal and 151 math. Although that is not stellar, it was enough to entice two schools to interview me.

Once you receive your GRE scores, you can then designate a few schools to send your scores to. You must use the correct code or your scores will not be sent to the schools of your choice. Some schools have a different code for their physician assistant program than the code for their actual school. I definitely ran into this problem and sent my scores to the correct school but not to the correct program and had to go back and pay more money to get my scores sent to the correct program.

And you must also designate the correct code for your CASPA application so that they can also receive your scores. You can find this code on the CASPA website. And this brings us to our next chapter entitled CASPA.

Chapter 5 - CASPA

So you've done the hard work. Now it's time for the annoying work. The CASPA is also known as the central application system for physician assistants. And it is very annoying. Not only do you have to go to all of your previous schools and have your transcripts sent to CASPA, you also have to enter all this information manually. Then someone cross references what you've entered with your transcripts. And they make any and all necessary corrections.

Once you've answered all of your information you also have to calculate your GPA, which is also corrected if you put it in wrong. Then you have to wait for your GRE scores to be sent to CASPA so they can verify what you've manually put in for your GRE score.

Depending on how many schools you've been to and how many classes you've taken, this could be a very tedious and monotonous process. I, for example, went to three schools, one of which I attended twice at two different times. So I had to enter all of my classes in year and semester order under each school. Not only do you have to enter your classes by correct name but also the grade you received. And again, if you enter the wrong class name, for example, "ethics applied" rather than "applied ethics", CASPA will automatically correct it.

CASPA also requires that you submit three letters of recommendation through their system. This means you have to enter the person's email address who is writing the letter of recommendation and their name and title so that CASPA can send that person an email explaining to them how they can submit their letter of recommendation.

Most of this is just waiting around for CASPA to receive all of your information. But you are still not done. You still also have to enter your work information, your volunteering information, your shadowing information, and any certifications or degrees that you received.

And finally, you get to have some fun. This is your essay that you submit through CASPA.

This is where you set yourself apart. You must write an amazing essay. But this is much easier than most people think. You don't have to write a bunch of fancy words or have complex sentences. All you need to do is show that you have empathy, compassion, and personality. Your essay must be compelling and show why they should pick you as a physician assistant. It must also prove that being a physician assistant is the only career for you.

And how do you do this?

That's easy. Tell a story, that's it. Don't write a formal essay like you are writing a research paper for class. Make this your story. Tell a story about how you had an experience one time going to an emergency room and interacting with a physician assistant either as a patient or as a person giving support to a patient. Make sure it's emotional and heartfelt. You want the person reading your essay to feel happy and smile, to feel sad and even cry, but do not leave them the way they were before they read your essay. You absolutely must emotionally affect the person who is reading your essay.

Tip: Write your essay as a generic essay. Do not address a single school. Sign off on your essay like the following: "Thank you for considering me for your Physician Assistant program. And when I am admitted, I promise that I will be the best PA that I can possible be. Sincerely, Nathaniel Dryden"

In my essay, I described the story that I told you earlier in this book. I also described how I dislocated my elbow in 11th grade. And I described when my father was diagnosed with stage IV non-small cell adenocarcinoma of the lung; lung cancer. He was a smoker all his life. And one day he called me complaining that he had been dizzy and had headaches for like six months and they were getting worse and worse. He was taking 20 goodie powders a day to no avail. I was driving when I received this phone call. I had to pull over and I told him with a stern and direct voice to go to the doctor. It still took him a few weeks before he finally listened to me. But by then it was too late. The doctors found the cancer but also discovered that the cancer had spread to his brain. There was nothing they could do for him. But they decided to do chemo and radiation anyway.

The story continues and yes, I added all this to my essay. It is true and it takes the reader on emotional ride. I also go on to say how I chose to be a physician assistant because of my previous experience and all my further experiences helped me to realize how personable physician assistants are and how they actually treat you like a human being instead of just a sickness. It does not matter how long or short your essay is, just as long as it is complete. But do remember, the faculty staff members who are reading your essay have tons of essays to read. So if you can make your point in less words, please do so. And make sure that you do not bash any other profession while you are talking up physician assistants.

And this brings me to the interview during which one of my interviewers challenged a statement I made about physicians and physician assistants.

Chapter 6 – Interview

So you've made it this far. And you have been granted an invite for an interview. How this works is you get an email saying that you have been selected to interview. You then have to click on a link and register for an interview on a particular day and time. Obviously, if your school is out of state or far enough away, you will have to make arrangements for a hotel, possibly an air flight, and a rental car. Do not miss your interview date.

Before you go to the interview there are few things that you need to know. The first thing is how to dress. Men should dress in a full suit with a tie and dress shoes. Women should wear either a business suit or a dress with heels. Women should remember to also bring a jacket of some sort if she decides to wear a dress just in case it is cold. You do not want to have a bad interview just because you are not comfortable.

Once you have figured out what you're going to wear during your interview, the next step is to practice your interview. There are many websites on the Internet with practice questions for your PA interview. Some weird ones that you may get go like this: "What animal would you be?" Or ethical questions like this: "If you had the choice to save your own child or group of people, which would you choose?"

I was lucky in the fact that I did not get any either of these types of questions. The most common types of questions, like the ones I got, are: Why do you want to be a PA? What is the difference between a PA and an NP? Why did you not go to Med school? Why did you choose our school? And general questions about you and your academic career.

Is also a good idea to prepare before your interview just like you did before the GRE. You want to make the day of your interview as stress-free as possible.

When I first arrived at my first interview, I parked in the parking lot and sat my car for a few minutes. This interview can be an anxiety provoking activity. But if you are prepared, you can minimize the nervousness that you feel.

When I first walked into the door there was a greeter who welcomed me and other interviewees. They ushered us into this room where they have what is called a meet and greet. During this meeting, they have snacks and drinks and allow you about 15 to 20 minutes just to walk around and meet everybody and shake hands. Some of the faculty also come in and talk to you. This 15 to 20 minutes is designed to get you comfortable. And it is a good amount of time to practice talking to people that you do not know and becoming more comfortable with it in this setting.

Next the interview coordinator comes in and tells you what your schedule will be. They grab you one by one to interview with the professors. In the meantime, the rest of the interviewees are either chaperoned or sit together and are allowed to mingle.

During my experience, before the interview, we were given a tour of the campus by two current students. The campus was fairly small, just one building. The two students showed us the classroom that we will be sitting in, the lab room where they also have a ping-pong table, the break room which has a refrigerator, a microwave, the lockers, and a pool table. And we were also shown the computer room where we would be taking our tests. These rooms were all on the second floor except for the exam room which was on the first floor.

After the tour, we were ushered into a single room where we had to write an essay. The essay was pretty open ended. In fact it was completely free write. We had to answer the question, "Why do you want to be a PA?"

And then we were escorted into another room and we were allowed to just chill while we were called one by one to interview with two professors. Sometimes the school will have each professor interview a student one on one and the students will rotate. Some schools will sit you at a long table with three or four professors for the interview.

The key here is to understand that they know that you will be nervous. But being nervous does not mean that you won't be able to handle yourself. And they will ask challenging questions just to see how you react. This is because PA school was very challenging and they need to know that you can handle the pressure.

I sat waiting for my interview speaking with the other prospective students. They brought us in one by one for the interview. When my name was called, I had a note pad, a pen, and a bottle of water. Then they sat me down at the end of the table, and the two professors sat on either side of me about two seats away.

They asked me how I was and we chitchatted for a few seconds before the real questions started. I sat back in my chair with my left arm resting on the back of the chair in my right arm, with pen in hand, resting on the table. Think of more of a relaxed, attentive look rather than an uncaring look.

They asked me the usual questions such as why I wanted to be a physician assistant rather than a nurse practitioner, why I did not go to med school, and why I chose their particular school. Remember to research their school so you know something about it. Knowing what their first time pass rate on graduates who take the PANCE is because you are interviewing the school just as much as they are interview you.

Then they started to challenge me. Well, at least they wanted to challenge me. But I featured my negatives and brought up my flaws before they could. Earlier in my undergrad I had a very rough stretch for a semester. It was bad enough that I actually failed my Calculus class. The same semester I took organic chemistry and had to make a decision which one I wanted to pass. I did not need calculus so I decide to focus all my energies on organic chemistry. It took many hours a day of studying for biology is my strong suit, not chemistry. But I managed to squeeze by with a high C.

Before they could bring that up, I brought it up. I simply stated the fact that I was very good at bouncing back from adversity when they asked me the question what my greatest strength was. And then I expounded on this by telling them as they can see, I received an F in calculus. One of the professors replied, "Yeah, what's up with that?" I explained to them my situation and how crazy that semester was for me. And then went on to explain other situations that challenged me that I was able to learn from, bounce back from, and not give up.

Although they did not like the F, they were intrigued by my ability to not let it crush me and my willingness to put in long hours to bring up my GPA. They even asked me how many hours I intended to study while I was in PA school. My answer was simple, I said as many hours as it takes. They liked that answer.

They also asked me if I had applied to medical school. I told him that I hadn't and then told them that I preferred to become a PA because it seems like PAs treat patients more like a person. One of my interviewers took this as an insult to physicians. She challenged me with it. I waited until she was finished, and then I calmly explained myself by saying that I was not intending to badmouth physicians but simply explaining my experience as a patient. And that I understood that physicians were under a lot of time pressure to get patients in and out. And I also understood that PAs have to do that too and I am willing to make that sacrifice if I need to.

So be prepared to be challenged during your interview. But do not interrupt your interviewers. Let them finish and then calmly and collectively reply to them. Remember, you do not need to answer right away. You can pause and think about your answer. A lot of these questions are designed just to see how you react. Your facial expression and tone of voice say much more than the words that are coming out of your mouth. So make sure you do some practicing in front of the mirror as someone asks you uncomfortable questions and pay attention to how you react non-verbally.

After their interview, I was thanked and the interviewers told me that they would be getting in touch but for me to continue to shadow. This is because I did not have a letter of recommendation from a physician assistant and I had not shadowed many hours with a physician assistant. They did question me on this and I replied that since I work in a hospital, physicians were more readily available.

After this interview, I got another interview with another school. This one was a little bit different although they did have the meet and greet in the beginning. They interviewed us one on one and we rotated through three different professors. They also had a writing section which was much more challenging. This essay asked us a medical and biological question. I cannot recall exactly what the question was but it was along the lines of how did your body regulate your temperature and adjust your blood pressure. So needless to say, make sure you know a little bit about the human body before applying to physician assistant school.

I only applied to four schools. I got interviews at two and denied at the other two. One of the reasons why I did not get an interview with the other two is because I did not take a class that they were requiring. So I could've actually saved some money if I did not apply to them.

If you haven't noticed by now, neither my application nor my application process was flawless. Now I will explain to you what you need to do after you've interviewed.

Chapter 7 – Post Interview

Sometimes students are accepted right then and there during their interview. But most often that is not how it works.

For me, I was rejected from the school that gave me my second interview, and I was put on the waiting list for the first school. I was a little bit pissed because I felt like I aced the interview. But I had to accept it.

What I did next I believe had the biggest impact on me getting into the school. Since I was on the waiting list there was obviously something they liked about me and some things that they felt that I could improve on. Since they told me to go ahead and keep shadowing, I did that.

I set up another shadowing experience with a physician assistant at the hospital that I worked at 3 to 4 days a week. I did this in the morning before work. And then every week, I would fax in my updated shadowing hours. I also rotated through the physician assistants and had them write me extra letters of recommendation which I also faxed.

Soon I had 50 more shadowing hours and three more letters of recommendation which I had faxed into the school. I believe this had a huge impact. I also called once a week after my fax to make sure that they had received it and to let them know that I was very interested in attending their school.

It wasn't long before I received that very awesome phone call saying that I had gotten into the school. They said that my letter of acceptance is on the way and that they emailed me a packet that I would have to sign and email back. Then they emailed me another packet that had all the tasks that I had to do before my orientation day.

Unfortunately for me, I only had about 2 to 3 weeks to prepare for my orientation day and the first week of classes. This is because I got put on the waiting list and it took a long time to get accepted. Usually, if you are accepted, you are accepted months in advance which gives you plenty of time to complete all of your tasks.

One of the things that I had to do was to buy a medical terminology book and complete it.

So I'm recommending that you go ahead and buy a medical terminology book and complete it. That way you will already have it done. It is also good practice and a great foundation of knowledge because once you are in school, you hit the ground running.

I also had to get my medical equipment such as a stethoscope, a sphygometer, a reflex hammer, an eyechart, a tape measure, gloves, an eye specula, alcohol wipes, tongued oppressors, a penlight, an ophthalmoscope, and tuning forks. These I bought on Amazon. If you do not have any, you will have to purchase scrubs. I would wait to find out if the school requires a certain color.

Once you get all of your equipment ready you will then be prepare for your orientation. You do not need all this equipment for your orientation but you do need it for the first week. So you might as well go ahead and get it done because my classes started the very next week. The next step is to attend your orientation which will be explained in the bonus chapter.

Chapter 8 – Conclusion

Before we go on to the bonus chapter, let's recap what we have learned in this book. I have scattered my story throughout this book not only for entertainment purposes, but also to show you a real-world example of how this works.

First, you must do well during your undergraduate. If you do not, then you risk never making it to physician assistant school or taking forever to get there. Try to strive for a GPA of 3.5 or greater. Next, you need to make connections with physician assistants and other medical professionals. These connections will help you get your foot in the door and will teach you and show you the ropes. Then you must study for and get at least a 300 on the GRE exam. Then you must enter all your information in the CASPA website including your transcript information, your GRE scores, your letters of recommendation, and your all-important personal essay.

Then if you're lucky enough to get an interview, you must also prepare for that. Then I showed you what to do after your interview to ensure you get the best possible chance of being accepted.

Remember to also check online for additional resources. A simple Google search will reveal more than enough. As I mentioned before, the Princeton Review is the book that I used study for the GRE. And make sure you also look up information on the interview, what to expect during your GRE exam day experience, how to correctly enter your information on CASPA, and do your own research on your local physician assistants to pick the best ones to shadow. The information in the preceding sentence is beyond the scope of this book. This book is to tell you what to do step-by-step to ensure that you get into physician assistant school. But you must then take the steps and delve deep into them so that you can make the best of your opportunity and tailor the steps to your own personality.

This is a short book because it is concise. It is not full of a bunch of fluff and unneeded, unnecessary information. I do not believe in wasting time. PA school taught me to be a time manager. Well actually, time management is what is known as a misnomer. The key is to actually manage yourself.

Now I will tell you what it is going to be like as a physician assistant student.

Bonus – Life as a PA Student

As a bonus, I would like to explain how physician assistant school is going to start and be for the entire time you are there. I did not have this guidance so I did not know what to expect. But by reading this book, you will not have that excuse and you will be much more prepared than I was.

My orientation lasted two full days. It was pretty boring just like most orientations are. There's a lot of paperwork and a lot of people that want to talk to you. During one session, all of the students had to stand up, state their name, and tell a little something about themselves. I felt like I was in grammar school again.

I was also seated at a particular table with my designated advisor. There were about seven or eight other students who also had the same advisor who also sat at this table. We had to show our advisor our finished medical terminology book. There were roughly 65 total students in my class.

After the long drawn out boring orientation, we get to get measured for our future white coats and we get the chance to purchase our school lab uniforms. These uniforms for us were a school T-shirt and a pair of sweatpants with the school logo on them. Yes they were overpriced. But they did accept credit. The white coat, however, must be ordered online. I would wait to do this.

The first week of class was no joke. Our classes started at 8 o'clock in the morning and did not finish until 5 o'clock in the afternoon. This was Monday through Friday. I would recommend living as close to the campus as humanly possible.

When you get out of class the last thing you're going to want to do is study. But that's exactly what you need to do; from the FIRST day! Get in the habit of grabbing a quick bite to eat, maybe taking a 20 minute nap, and then getting right on to studying. I would say study until about no later than 11 o'clock. You will most definitely be sleep deprived.

Most students do not do much studying this first week of class. This is a mistake. The classes build on each other and the material does not slow down. You're in class 8 hours a day and only have roughly 4 hours to study that material. And everyone knows the golden rule of studying is to study two hours for every hour that you're in class. You will not be doing this in PA school.

But you do have the weekend to make up for any of the studying that you need to catch up on from the week. But make sure you do take some time off for yourself or you will burn out. Make sure you know a lot of learning techniques before you start studying for physician assistant school. Learn memorization techniques, word association, mnemonics, and many other ways that will help you memorize the material.

And know this, memorization is only half the battle. You must also be able to apply this information. You will be presented, on the exam, with scenarios and you must first diagnose the condition and then develop the treatment based on clues. Diagnosis and treatments start in your second semester. But the Anatomy and Physiology class in the first semester is a killer.

You will not have time to memorize all the material, so be smart with your time. The first exam for each professor counts but for you it's also a trial exam to learn how the professor asks his or her questions. So do not be too down on yourself if you do not do so hot on the first exams.

My school required a 75 in order to pass the exam. Your school may be a little different but I highly doubt that it will take anything less than a 70 to pass. And exams get progressively harder the further you get into PA school. You will have days when you have three on the computer exams, plus a lab practical, and a project to complete.

There will be literally days when you want to kill yourself. But these days and these weeks are manageable. Sometimes students run into a major anxiety problem and have to speak to a psychologist. If this happens to you be okay with it. Do whatever you have to do to get through the program. No one said that it would be easy. That is why passing physician assistant school is so rewarding. You have to learn pretty much everything a medical student learns and you have to learn it in roughly 27 months. Actually, it's less than that because 12 of those months are your rotations. So if you have to see a doctor to get medication while you are in PA school, then do not hesitate. I guarantee that at least half of your class will be on Adderall, Prozac, or some kind of anti-depressant. Just make sure you do this ethically and legally.

During PA school you will be eating quick, studying a lot, not sleeping well, you will have no social life, and you still have to balance in activities of daily life. Make sure you take advantage of your resources. Talk to your buddy (an upperclassman PA student will be assigned to you as your buddy), your fellow students, the PAs that you shadowed, and the faculty when you need help. And make sure that you are on top of things. Ask a professor to show you the equipment in the lab room when you start having to use it that way, when you have your exercises, you do not look like you do not know what you are doing.

Also, get to know your medical equipment before attending your first day of physician assistant school. Make sure you know how to charge your ophthalmoscope and how to use a stethoscope and a blood pressure cuff. Most of your learning is going to occur outside of class during your own time. When the professors are lecturing they do not stop. They go and talk nonstop for about two hours (with a 5-10 minute break between the hours). Then you get about a 10 to 15 minute break. And then another professor comes in and talks for another two hours. Then you get a half an hour lunch. And you get two more sections like the morning sections in the afternoon.

This schedule is Monday through Friday. Except for lab days and exam days, during which you spend half your day in the lab. And you usually have your lab practical on the same day as an exam day. So make sure you use your time outside of class to also practice what you are learning for your lab practical. There is not enough time in the lab itself to learn the techniques that you will be imploring during your lab practical's. The weekend comes in very handy. You will not have a social life outside of PA school. Your fellow physician assistant students will become your family, and your professors will as well.

You will fail at least one exam during your physician assistant educational career. So be prepared for that and expect it. But with three failures in one semester, you will have to go see what is called CSP. Basically you just meet with your advisor and other fellow faculty members and talk about what is going on. Every failure after that will also trigger you to have to go see CSP. If you get too many failures in one semester, they reserve the right to dismiss you from the class. But they often give you a chance to resign rather than to be dismissed so that it looks better on your transcript. But don't worry, that won't happen to you!

PA school is relentless and I tell you the information in the preceding paragraph not to scare you, but to prepare you.

Good luck with your physician assistant studies and I know you will be GREAT!

Author

Nathaniel Dryden

Connect with him on Twitter:
@NathanielDryden

You may tweet at the author if you have any questions, concerns, suggestions, or are in need for clarification. Do not be shy.

If you enjoyed this book and have found value in it, please leave feedback on the website from which you purchased it. Thank you and good luck with your education.

www.ingramcontent.com/pod-product-compliance
Lightning Source LLC
Chambersburg PA
CBHW021440170526
45164CB00001B/329